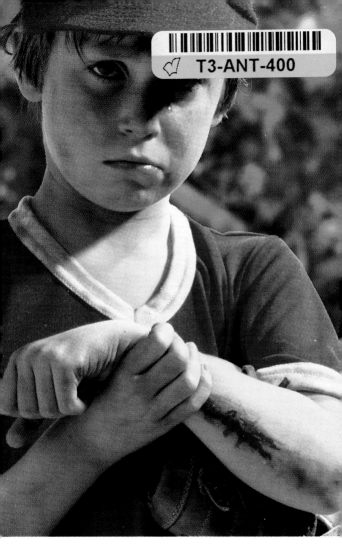

When infection takes hold, Neosporin* takes charge

Neosporin Cream
<u>Neosporin Ointment</u>
Prescribed so often
because it performs so well

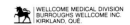

WELLCOME MEDICAL DIVISION
BURROUGHS WELLCOME INC.
KIRKLAND, QUÉ.

*Trade Mark

PAAB
CCPP

Pocket Picture Guides
to Clinical Medicine

Skin Diseases

Pocket Picture Guides
to Clinical Medicine

Skin Diseases

Denis E. Sharvill FRCP

Consultant Dermatologist, South East Kent,
Canterbury and Thanet Health Districts, UK

Williams & Wilkins Baltimore London

Western Hemisphere distribution rights held by
Williams and Wilkins
428 East Preston Street
Baltimore, MD 21202, USA

ISBN 0-683-07689-4 (Williams and Wilkins)
      0-906923-17-4 (Gower)

Library of Congress Cataloging in Publication Data
Sharvill, D.
    Skin diseases.
    (Pocket picture guides to clinical medicine)
    1. Skin – Diseases – Diagnosis – Atlases. I. Title.
II. Series. [DNLM: 1. Skin diseases – Diagnosis – Atlases.
WR 17 S532s]
RL105. S45 1984   616. 5'075   83-5843

Project Editor: Fiona Carr
      Designer: Teresa Foster

Originated in Hong Kong by Imago Publishing Ltd.
Printed in Great Britain by W. S. Cowell Ltd.

Pocket Picture Guides
to Clinical Medicine

The purpose of this series is to provide essential visual
information about commonly encountered diseases in a
convenient practical and economic format. Each Pocket
Picture Guide covers an important area of day-to-day
clinical medicine. The main feature of these books is the
superbly photographed color reproductions of typical
clinical appearances. Other visual diagnostic
information, such as X-rays, is included where
appropriate. Each illustration is fully explained by a
clearly written descriptive caption highlighting important
diagnostic features. Tables presenting other diagnostic
and differential diagnostic information are included
where appropriate. A comprehensive and carefully
compiled index makes each Pocket Picture Guide an easy
to use source of visual reference.

An extensive series is planned and other titles in the
initial group of Pocket Picture Guides are:

Infectious Diseases
Rheumatic Diseases
Sexually Transmitted Diseases
Pediatrics

Pr *Cicatrin**

POWDER / CREAM 15 g

*To eradicate
bacteria
and promote
re-epithelialization
without touching
the wounds.*

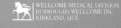

WELLCOME MEDICAL DIVISION
BURROUGHS WELLCOME INC
KIRKLAND, QUE.

*Trade Mark

Contents

Introduction

The skin is a very large organ, subject to many diseases. Most of the diseases seen in a community are of a few common types, but these will differ from country to country. Many conditions are rare and are only of academic interest to the specialist. Some, however, although not very common, are important, either because they are dangerous in themselves, or because they point to some important general illness.

This small pocket book makes no attempt to cover the whole of dermatology, but rather to illustrate pictorially some diagnostic points which have seemed important to the author in hospital practice in England. It must be realised that many common skin conditions are subtle in appearance and therefore difficult to photograph and to reproduce in print. Conversely, the temptation to include uncommon or unimportant conditions which make attractive pictures has been avoided.

Selection of material is, therefore, idiosyncratic, but it is hoped that this collection will prove useful in the differential diagnosis of skin diseases which may appear superficially very similar.

Eczema-dermatitis

The terms eczema and dermatitis are used synonymously in British dermatology. The classification of eczema and its aetiology are not discussed here.

Endogenous eczema

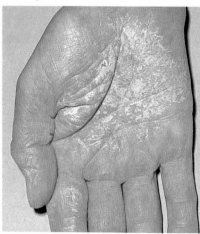

Fig. 1 Chronic hypertrophic eczema of the palm. This may be constitutional or due to friction or long-standing irritation. It may be difficult to distinguish from psoriasis (see Fig. 41).

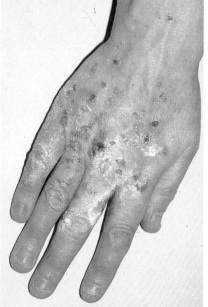

Fig. 2 Acute exacerbation of chronic atopic eczema which has been much excoriated.

1

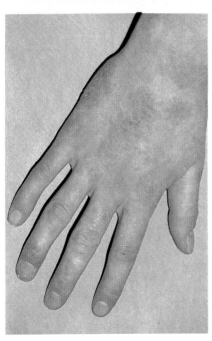

Fig. 3 Chronic dry eczema on the back of the hand of the type often seen in housewives or in any dry-skinned patients who are subjected to water, solvents etc.

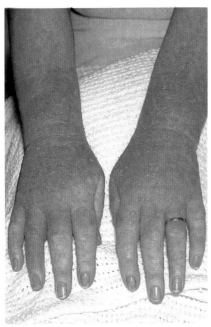

Fig. 4 Acute eczematous dermatitis of both hands and forearms which suggests a contact cause, perhaps rubber gloves.

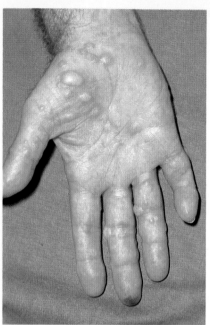

Fig. 5 Vesicular eczema of the type often called pompholyx, for which, frequently, no cause can be found. Attacks may be recurrent over many years.

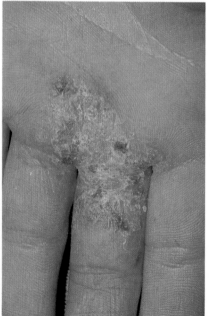

Fig. 6 Localised patch of crusted and infected eczema in an atopic child. Such patches responded readily to treatment but recurred over many months.

3

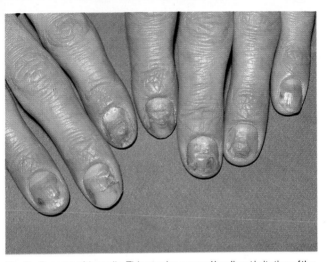

Fig. 7 Eczema of the nails. This may be caused by direct irritation of the nails or, as in this case, can be secondary to chronic eczema of the fingers. The nails themselves show transverse ridging and discoloration, which is characteristic of eczema. The diagnosis of all nail conditions is extremely difficult; this case could be mistaken for fungal infection or even for psoriasis.

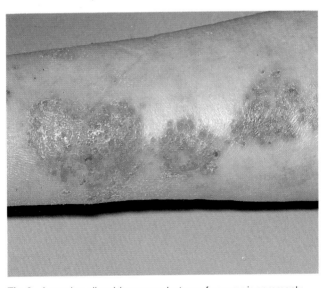

Fig. 8 An oozing, discoid or nummular type of eczema is commonly seen on the forearms and legs, running a chronic course over months or years. Although suppressive treatment is fairly successful in this sort of eczema, a cause can seldom be found.

4

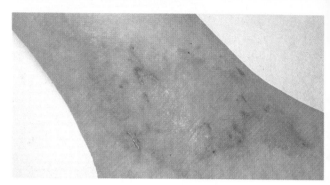

Fig. 9 Chronic excoriated and lichenified eczema of the ankle. This type of eczema is often termed neurodermatitis and is perpetuated by scratching or as here by rubbing one foot against the other leg.

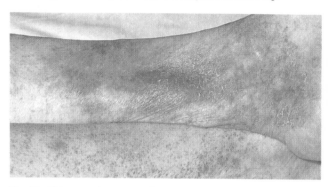

Fig. 10 This case of eczema at first appears similar to the example above, but shows chronic hypostatic pigmentation which is often wrongly called varicose eczema. It can occur in the absence of varicose veins although it does indicate circulatory deficiency of some kind.

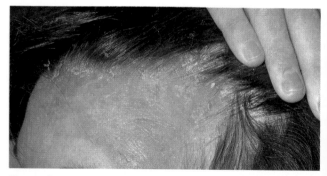

Fig .11 Seborrhoeic dermatitis of the forehead and scalp. It may be difficult, often impossible, to distinguish this from psoriasis (see Fig. 39).

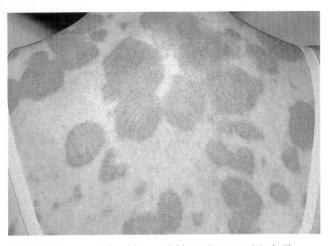

Fig. 12 Widespread discoid or petaloid eruption associated with seborrhoeic dermatitis at other sites. This cleared up rapidly with simple treatment which it would not have done if it had been psoriasis.

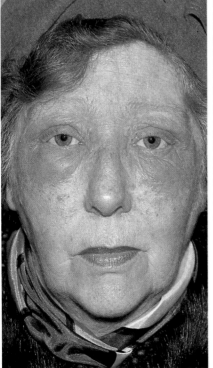

Fig. 13 Eczematous eruptions around the eyes and on the face generally can be extremely difficult to treat. Cosmetics are frequently blamed but are seldom the cause. It may be worthwhile to investigate such cases using patch testing. Active ingredients and preservatives in eye medications can cause this sort of rash and allergic sensitivity to nail varnish commonly produces a rash on the sides of the neck or on the eyelids.

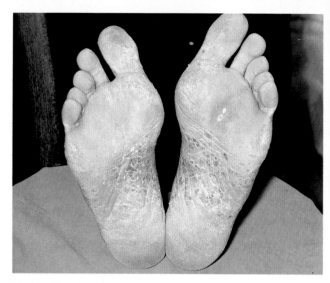

Fig. 14 Chronic vesico-pustular eczema of the central soles. This is frequently wrongly diagnosed as tinea pedis, which is not a differential diagnosis. Some dermatologists refer to all cases of this type as either pustular psoriasis, chronic palmar plantar pustulosis, recalcitrant eruption of the palms and soles, bacterid etc. Such cases are difficult to treat.

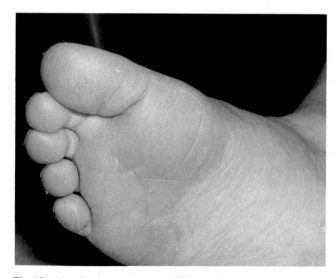

Fig. 15 Juvenile plantar dermatosis. This condition is associated with the wearing of modern non-porous footwear and has only appeared in dermatological literature in relatively recent years.

Infantile eczema

Eczema may begin at any age and in children it may cause parental concern about prognosis. In babies it is often mild and transient, yielding to simple treatment.

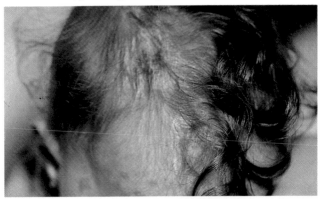

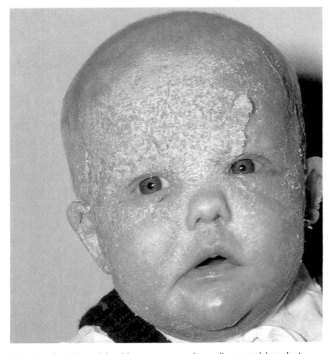

Fig. 16 'Cradle cap' (top) is common and usually no problem, but sometimes it persists and spreads to the face (bottom), indicating the beginning of atopic eczema.

8

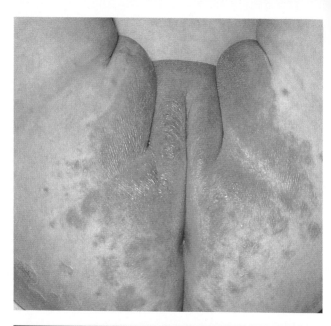

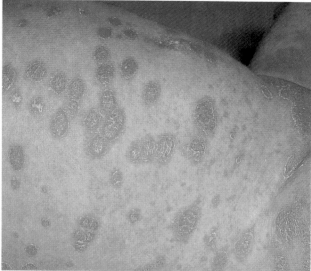

Fig. 17 Napkin rashes are commonly due to low grade infection under infrequently changed, occlusive plastic pants. This rash at first appeared to be a simple nappy rash (top), but spread (bottom) and resembled psoriasis. This type of infantile eczema looks alarming, but responds to treatment and may have a good long-term prognosis.

9

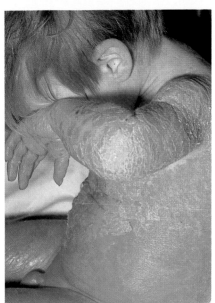

Fig. 18 The appearance of widespread, severe infantile atopic eczema with its attendant misery is unmistakable. The immediate prognosis in hospital is good, but the outcome is less certain. It is easy to make statistical statements about prognosis based on hospital figures, but much more difficult to assess an individual infant.

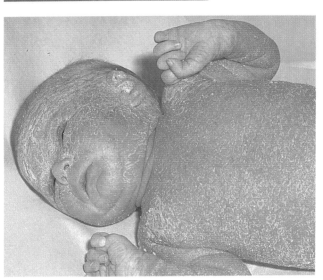

Fig. 19 Most persistent atopic eczema produces dryness and lichenification. Some infants present from the beginning with dry skin which they scratch incessantly. It is sometimes difficult to decide whether this is primary atopic eczema, or eczema secondary to ichthyosis. A careful history and follow-up usually determines the cause, but both conditions may coexist, as here.

10

Contact dermatitis

This may be caused by irritation or allergic sensitivity and is a vast subject which can only be summarised very briefly. Occasionally the diagnosis is obvious but often it demands painstaking investigation by patch testing, visiting places of work etc. Many cases of contact dermatitis are due to medication.

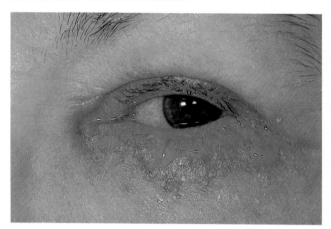

Fig. 20 This patient had a mild conjunctivitis which was treated with neomycin ointment. When this proved ineffective she was given soframycin which made the condition worse; however it settled quickly after withdrawing antibiotics.

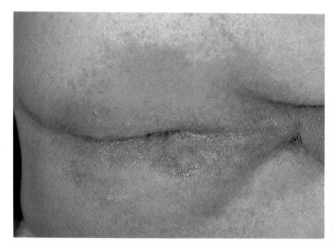

Fig. 21 Proprietary haemorrhoid ointments contain multiple sensitising ingredients. This particular dermatitis was caused by cinchocaine.

11

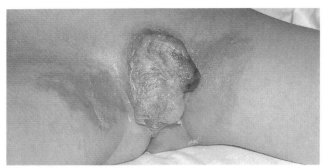

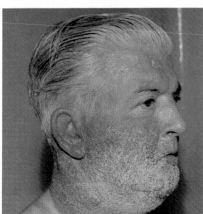

Fig. 22 Severe dermatitis can be caused by sensitivity to cetrimide. This child (above) was prescribed 1% cetrimide lotion which produced this violent reaction. The man on the left has a rash caused by cetrimide being used as an antiseptic before a face wound was sutured.

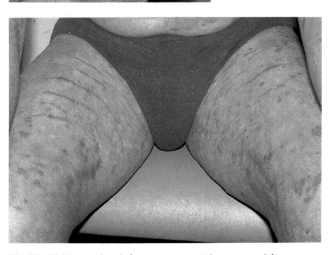

Fig. 23 Widespread and often permanent striae can result from applying strong steroids for psoriasis, as here.

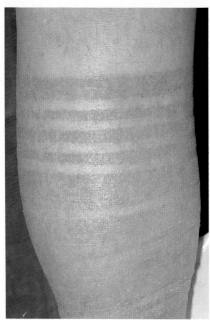

Fig. 24 Dermatitis from sticking plaster is common and zinc oxide plasters are used less frequently as a result. This patient was sensitised to the dye in a ventilated diachylon paste leg bandage, rather than the adhesive.

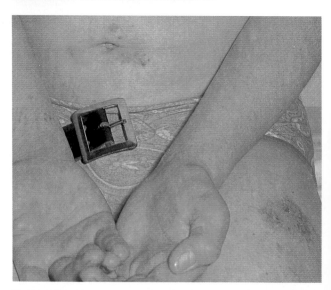

Fig. 25 Nickel in women and chromium in men are common causes of dermatitis. Suspenders, costume jewellery and coins may initiate dermatitis in women. This boy showed a reaction to the buckle of his belt, his wrist-watch strap and coins carried in his trouser pocket.

13

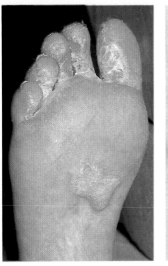
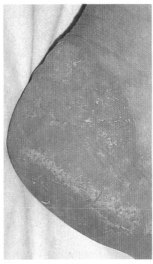

Fig. 26 Rubber is a frequent cause of dermatitis. This girl was diagnosed as having athlete's foot, which only rarely looks like this (compare Fig. 154). The condition of the heels (right) should have made the diagnosis clear, as a reaction to footwear.

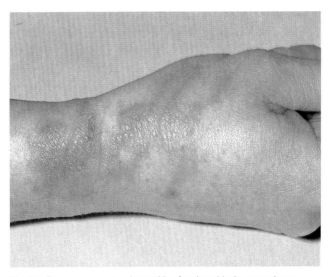

Fig.27 Plants may cause dermatitis of various kinds, sometimes consisting of non-specific erythma and redness, often in explosive attacks on the face. Sometimes where there is actual contact with the plant, peculiar linear and blistering eruptions may occur and this may be associated with light sensitivity as in phyto-photo-dermatitis.

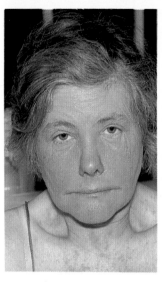
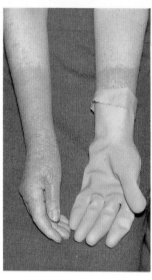

Fig.28 Occupational dermatitis is occasionally obvious but may be very difficult to diagnose. This lady, a cleaner, complained of a rash on her face, however, it was found that her rash was due to wearing rubber gloves, and as soon as she stopped using them she recovered.

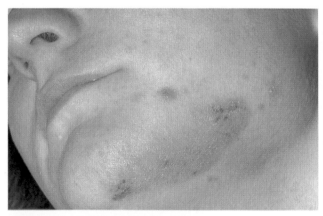

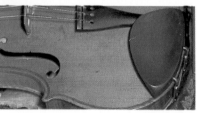

Fig. 29 The cause of this dermatitis was a reaction to the patient's violin chin-rest. Treatment, however, proved exceedingly difficult and she had to give up playing the violin.

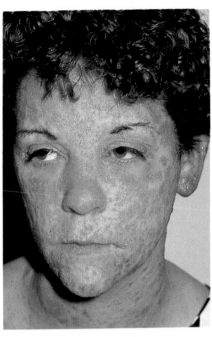

Fig. 30 Cosmetics are often unjustly blamed for causing facial dermatitis, although most dermatologists see many patients reacting to hair dyes containing p-phenylene diamine or related chemicals. This dermatitis commonly affects the ears and eyes, and in this case the whole face, rather than the scalp itself.

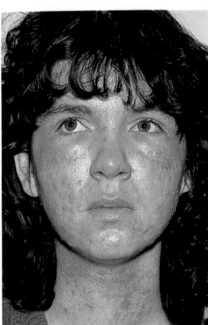

Fig. 31 This patient had suffered several attacks of explosive and severe dermatitis of her face. Previous attacks had been shown to be due to a cosmetic. After 50 patch tests she showed allergic sensitivity to an antiseptic and an emulsifier used in the cosmetic and an irritant reaction to propylene glycol.

16

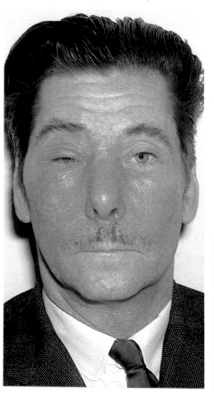

Fig. 32 An erythematous and oedematous reaction on the face and thigh. This is due to the chemical phosphorus sesquisulphide contained in the heads of 'strike anywhere' matches. Particles discharged into the air affected the patient's face.

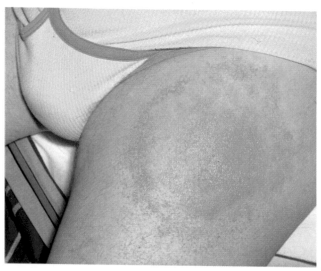

Psoriasis and Lichen Planus

Psoriasis

Psoriasis is a common condition affecting more than 1% of the population in Western countries. The typical patches of the knees and elbows are so well known to all doctors that they need not be illustrated.

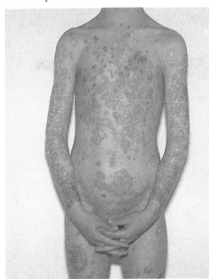

Fig. 33 Acute psoriasis in a child following an attack of tonsillitis. Sometimes this type of psoriasis presents difficulties in diagnosis and may be mistaken for a reaction to the drug used for treating the sore throat.

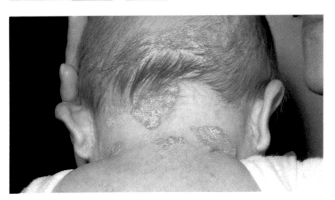

Fig. 34 Psoriasis is thought to be rare in babies and very young children although there is still debate as to whether the psoriasis-like eruption which sometimes occurs in babies is the fore-runner of psoriasis later on. The rash in this baby looked very like psoriasis but cleared up in two weeks and did not recur during the following year, which would be unusual in adult psoriasis of this type.

18

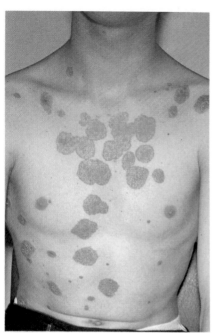

Fig. 35 Eruptive discoid psoriasis in a young man of 16 years (compare Fig. 12).

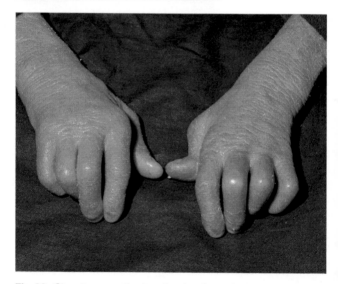

Fig. 36 Chronic generalised erythrodermic psoriasis with multiple joint involvement. This patient had had his finger joints replaced but was still severely disabled in spite of many systemic treatments such as methotrexate.

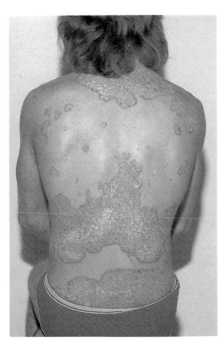

Fig. 37 Widespread plaque psoriasis. This sort of psoriasis is a devastating social handicap. It can usually be cleared quickly with conventional treatment as an in-patient, or systemic treatment may be used in spite of some degree of risk.

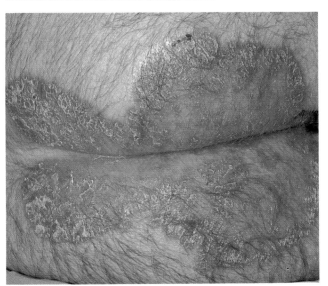

Fig. 38 Psoriasis in the flexures is not always as obvious as in this case and sometimes presents only as erythema and itching. Early diagnosis is important as treatment may be prolonged and difficult.

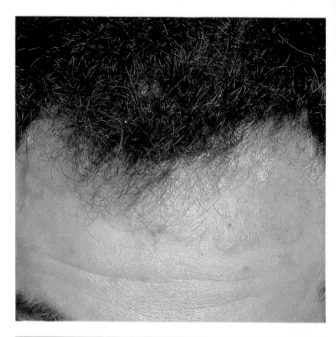

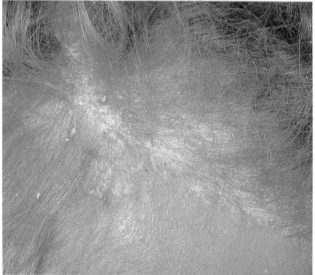

Fig. 39 Psoriasis of the scalp and hairline may closely resemble seborrhoeic dermatitis (top; compare Fig. 11) or may present a chronic scaly appearance often with localised discs in the scalp (bottom).

21

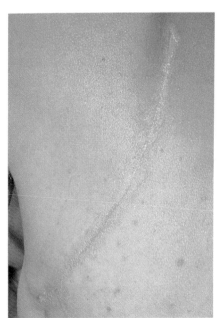

Fig. 40 Psoriasis is one of the conditions which may exhibit Koebner's isomorphic phenomenon. This is also seen in lichen planus (see Fig. 46). In this instance it occurred shortly after the healing of a surgical wound.

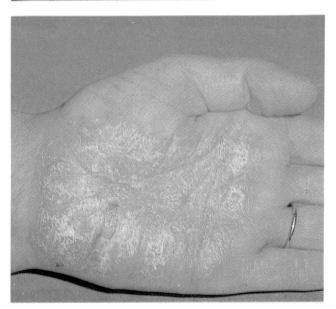

Fig. 41 Psoriasis may be limited to the palms and soles. Note the resemblance to chronic hypertrophic eczema of the palms (see Fig. 1).

22

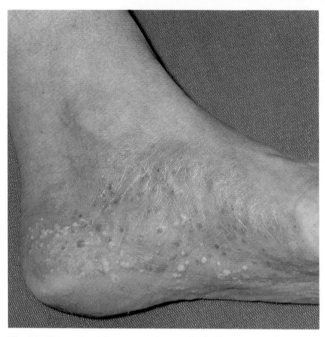

Fig. 42 This patient shows pustular psoriasis. Note how it affects the heel and the inner sole – areas seldom attacked by fungal infection.

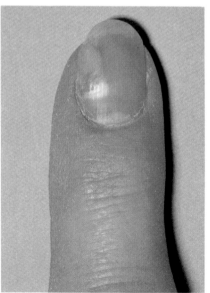

Fig. 43 Onycholytic type of nail involvement. Very similar appearances may be seen in infection, particularly with *Candida*, as a result of trauma or for no apparent reason.

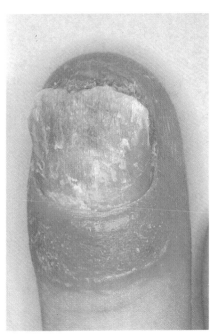

Fig. 44 Chronic thickening of the nail due to psoriasis, with involvement of the distal joint of the thumb (left). Psoriatic nails may also show thimble-like pitting (below) – this appearance can be seen in conditions other than psoriasis.

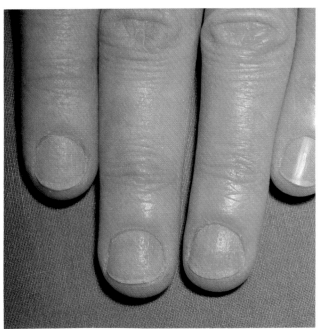

24

Lichen planus

Lichen planus is another common dermatosis of uncertain aetiology and nearly always causes confusion to the non-specialist. Clues may be given by the distribution, particularly over the anterior wrists, shins and lumbo-sacral area, often with involvement of the mucous membranes. Itching is also usually a feature but may be absent, and the distribution may be atypical. Careful examination in a good light will usually show at least a few of the typical lichen planus papules although the rest of the rash may look non-specific.

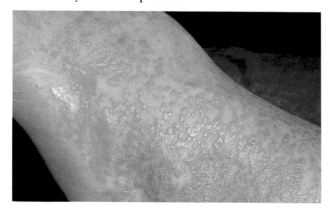

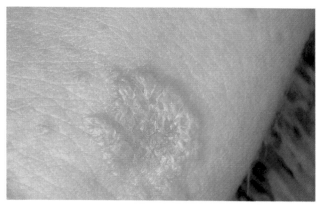

Fig. 45 Lichen planus papules tend to be polygonal rather than circular, and flat-topped rather than rounded. They have a very characteristic colour which is sometimes said to resemble lilac or violets. Papules also tend to be shiny when viewed by oblique light, and close examination will often show a milky white reticular appearance called Wickham's striae (bottom).

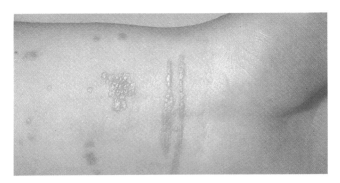

Fig. 46 Typical lesions on the wrist including Koebner's phenomenon (see Fig. 40).

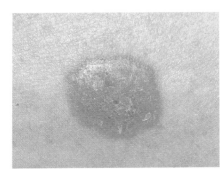

Fig. 47 An individual large papule of lichen planus. Sometimes a patient will show no more than one or two such lesions.

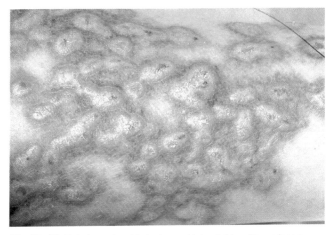

Fig. 48 Multiple hypertrophic lesions which might well have been diagnosed as lichenified eczema or nodular prurigo. The patient had, however, previously suffered from eruptive lichen planus and these lesions still showed lichen planus histology.

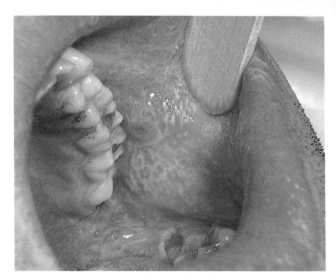

Fig. 49 Characteristic reticular appearance of the buccal mucous membrane which needs to be distinguished from simple thickening along the occlusal line and from premalignant leukoplakia.

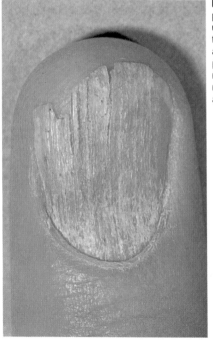

Fig. 50 Lichen planus may rather uncommonly affect the nails and produce atrophy. It has a bad prognosis and the nails seldom grow normally once affected.

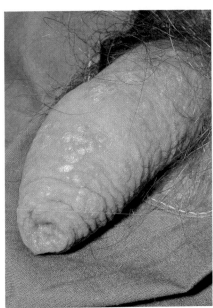

Fig. 51 The penis is a characteristically affected site, and may arouse fears of venereal disease. Secondary syphilis may present with a rash closely resembling lichen planus, but usually does not itch.

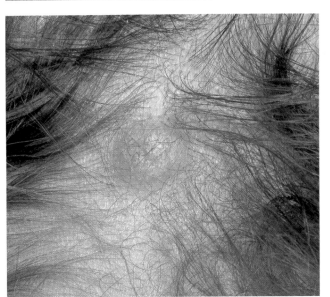

Fig. 52 Lichen planus does not often affect the scalp, but when it does, cicatricial and permanent alopecia may result. The end result of this condition is more commonly seen as multiple small, shiny, bald patches usually under 1cm in diameter.

28

Congenital and Naevoid Conditions

There are many types of localised or generalised birth marks, or naevi, and numerous genodermatoses, but many of these are extremely rare and are of interest only to the paediatric dermatologist or to the parents of the affected child.

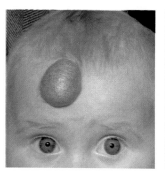
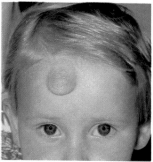

Fig. 53 Common strawberry naevus or cavernous haemangioma. This may cause parental alarm but always involutes with the passage of time (right), although sometimes minor surgical tidying-up is necessary.

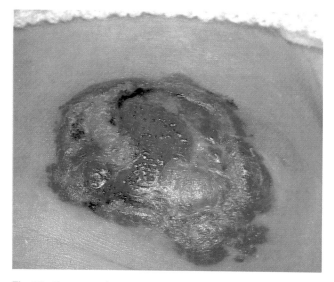

Fig. 54 Even a very large cavernus haemangioma, such as here on the breast of a baby girl, is probably better left alone, although over the years there have been changes in treatment and some now advocate laser treatment.

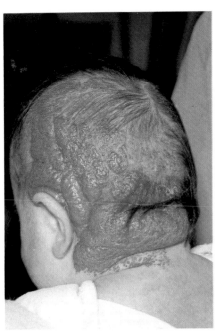

Fig. 55 A giant haemangioma of the scalp in a baby who died shortly afterwards with multiple vascular abnormalities inside the skull.

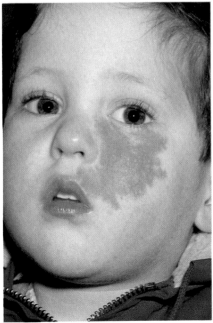

Fig. 56 Capillary haemangioma – port wine stain. These do not disappear and at present there is no satisfactory treatment other than cosmetic camouflage.

30

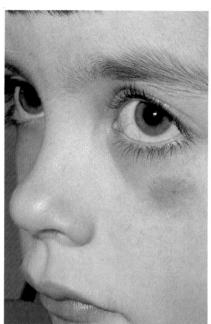

Fig. 57 Spider naevus. These are common in children and may erupt in women during pregnancy. They are easily treated by cauterising the central vessel.

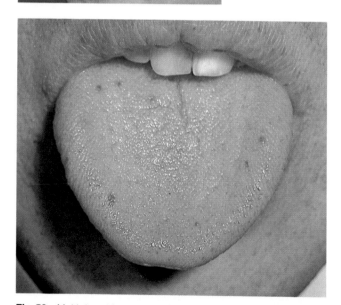

Fig. 58 Multiple spider naevi on the tongue and lips may indicate, as here, Osler's hereditary telangiectasia which may be of serious significance in case of haemorrhage.

31

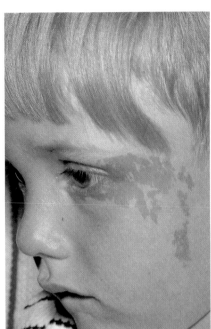

Fig. 59 Pigmented naevus on the face. These naevi occur in all shapes and sizes and are not amenable to treatment.

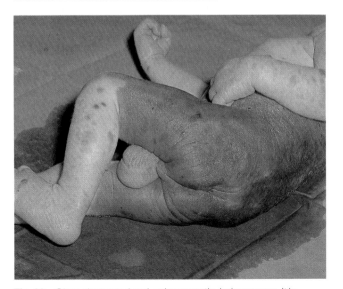

Fig. 60 Giant pigmented and, subsequently, hairy naevus. It is recommended that such gigantic lesions be removed because of the likelihood of malignant change later in life. Fortunately such lesions are very rare.

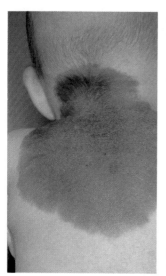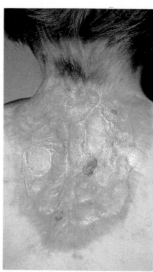

Fig. 61 Large pigmented naevus (left) and the result of plastic surgery (right). This emphasises that plastic surgeons are not magicians and can not undertake major repairs of this sort without leaving a scar.

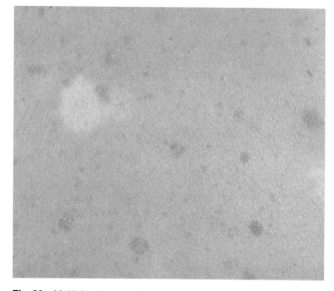

Fig. 62 Multiple pigmented naevi on the trunk including halo naevi. These often cause parental concern but do not need active intervention.

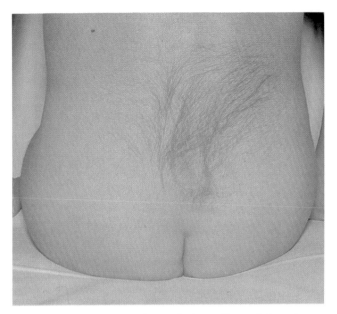

Fig. 63 Hairy naevus, sometimes called sacral fawn tail. Sometimes these lesions are associated with abnormalities of the underlying spine which should always be examined radiologically. Surgical treatment in time may prevent subsequent neurological damage if diastematomyelia is present.

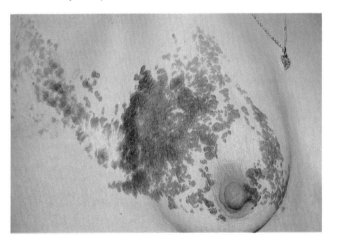

Fig. 64 Extensive pigmented warty naevus on the breast and flank of a young woman. Plastic surgeons could offer no treatment, but over the course of several years the whole of the naevus was removed by piecemeal destruction with a liquid nitrogen spray.

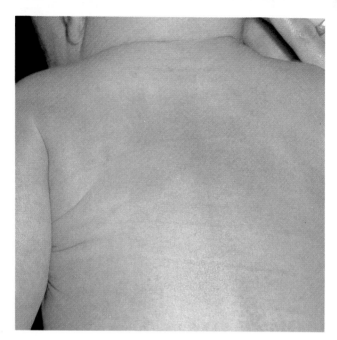

Fig. 65 Mongolian blue spot. This has no association with mongolism or Down's syndrome and although it may alarm the parents it disappears spontaneously. Care should be taken to differentiate this condition from bruising in cases of suspected child abuse.

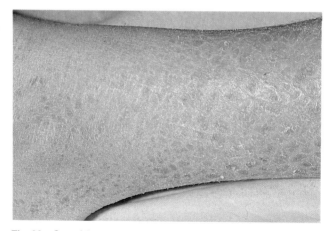

Fig. 66 One of the many varieties of congenital ichthyosis or dry skin which is usually most easily seen on the lower outer leg. There are so many different types of ichthyosis, varying from mild to life-destroying, that it is not possible to illustrate them all.

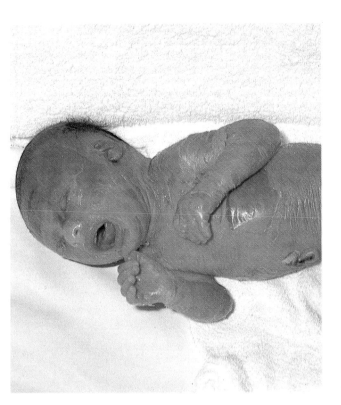

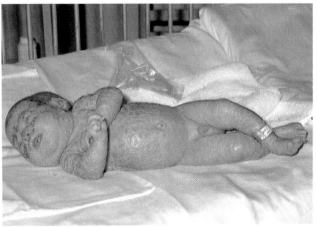

Fig. 67 Above: Baby with congenital ichthyosiform erythroderma. Below: The same baby a few weeks later. The erythroderma has disappeared and he shows a dry, scaly appearance.

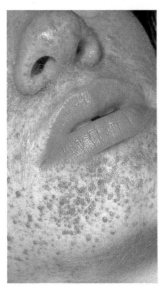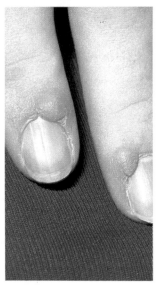

Fig. 68 An example of the condition known as adenoma sebaceum. This is not an adenoma and has nothing to do with the sebaceous apparatus, but it is important as an indicator of epiloia with its potentially serious complications. These patients may also have characteristic periungual fibromata (right).

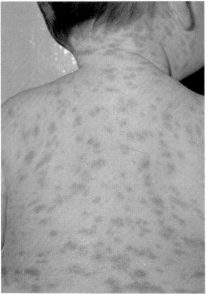

Fig. 69 Urticaria pigmentosa or mastocytosis which presents in small babies as these characteristic brownish macules which urticate on rubbing and often disappear around puberty.

37

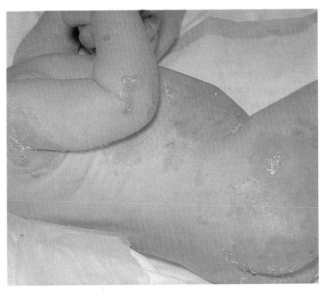

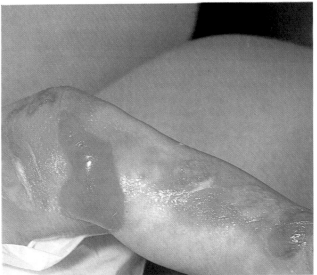

Fig. 70 Two of the many varieties of epidermolysis bullosa. Some of these are trivial and benign, others are life-threatening or life-destroying. Bullous diseases in the new-born constitute a complex diagnostic problem and infection is a much more common cause of blistering than these rare congenital abnormalities. The bullous disorders of the adult may occur in childhood, but not in small babies. The term pemphigus neonatorum now has little significance.

38

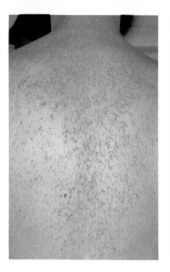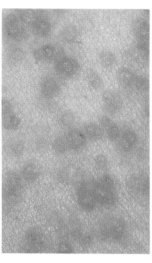

Fig. 71 Darier's disease - keratosis follicularis. This is an uncommon condition and is only included because effective treatment is now sometimes available in the form of the retinoid substance etretinate. Untreated, the condition can be so unpleasant as to make life almost intolerable or indeed it may be a danger to life. Some patients can now be given a large measure of relief or even complete remission.

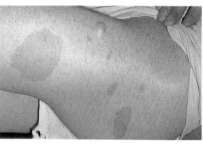

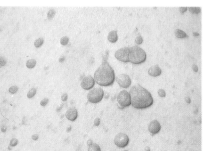

Fig. 72
Neurofibromatosis or von Recklinghausen's disease. Various forms of café au lait patches, neurofibromata and soft skin lesions may occur and, as the condition may run in families, genetic counselling may be necessary. Often it does not appear until adolescence or early adult life, and it is not entirely harmless. Intracranial lesions may occur, such as acoustic neuroma and sometimes the lesions undergo malignant transformation.

Miscellaneous Dermatoses

Acne vulgaris

Acne vulgaris is so common that it scarcely needs illustrating and its management is usually straightforward.

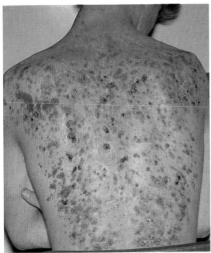

Fig. 73 A fulminating form of cystic and pustular acne which is actually ulcerating. Unless treated urgently and vigorously this will cause permanent scarring and disfigurement.

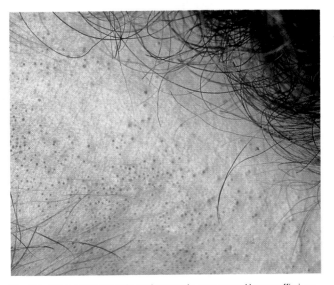

Fig. 74 These blackheads on the temple are caused by paraffin in a cosmetic.

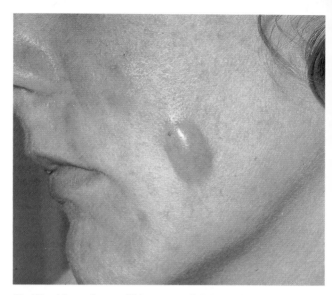

Fig. 75 A form of acne with large superficial cysts. These do not respond to ordinary remedies and may be followed by unpleasant scarring if incised. They usually respond readily to intralesional steroid injections.

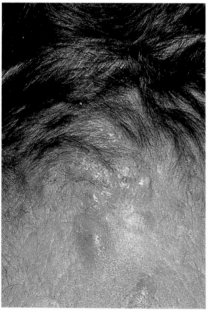

Fig. 76 Acne keloid seen on the back of the neck. It usually occurs quite apart from ordinary acne vulgaris and is resistant to treatment.

41

Rosacea

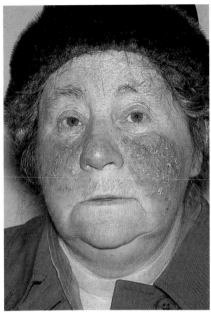

Fig. 77 Rosacea is a common condition and is easily treated. Such patients are, however, frequently referred to hospitals as examples of acute systemic lupus erythematosus, although the characteristic butterfly rash of that condition is very rare and is always associated with severe systemic illness. There are, however, many border-line cases of rosacea in which the diagnosis is difficult and which may be confused with contact dermatitis or erysipelas.

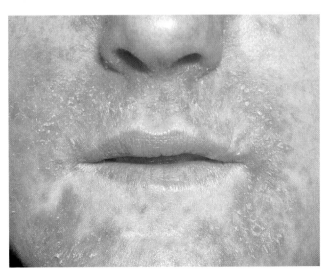

Fig. 78 Perioral dermatitis. This is a condition of relatively recent description occurring in a younger age group than rosacea, and separate from acne vulgaris. Many cases are certainly initiated by the injudicious use of steroids in banal skin conditions of the face.

Ulcerated legs

Ulcerated legs are common and tend to be regarded as a nuisance because their treatment is time consuming.

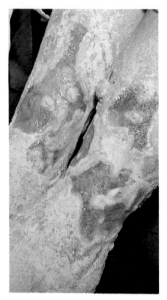

Fig. 79 Extensive bilateral post-thrombotic ulceration of the legs, of 20 years duration. The patient had never been treated adequately before, but the legs healed in less than three months with firm compression bandaging.

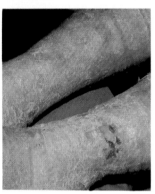

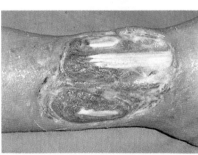

Fig. 80 This patient was also treated by compression bandaging treatment in out-patients.

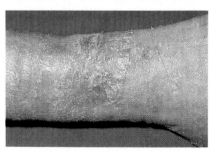

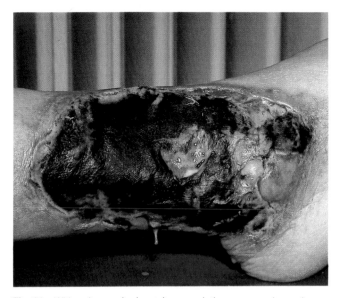

Fig. 81 With an increasingly ageing population, more and more leg ulcers are arterial in origin, or arterial deficiency supervenes in what were originally venous ulcers. This patient has an arterial ulcer of rapid onset. After being cleared in hospital a skin graft was successful but broke down soon afterwards.

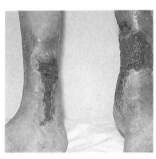

Fig. 82 The unusual causes of leg ulcers are so numerous that they cannot be listed here, but they should always be borne in mind as they may require different or specific forms of treatment. These are leg ulcers in a patient with spherocytosis. They healed after splenectomy.

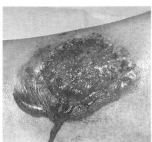

Fig. 83 An ulcer in a patient suffering from pyoderma gangrenosum. Several such ulcers occurred over a period of months and the patient was found to be suffering from ulcerative colitis.

44

Benign and Malignant Tumours of the Skin

Benign tumours

Most people suffer from lumps and bumps in their skin, at some time or another and have a number of pigmented or non-pigmented moles which can be regarded as harmless.

Sometimes warts present diagnostic problems, for example the flat warts seen on the face and hands of the young, or sometimes the mosaic warts of the feet.

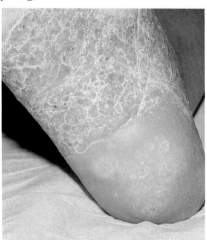

Fig. 84 This patient was unfortunate enough to have two intractable conditions, namely multiple plantar warts on the heel and chronic pustular psoriasis of the central foot.

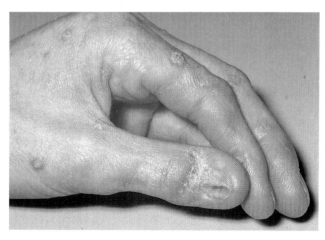

Fig. 85 This patient's warts were still flourishing 15 years after radiotherapy which caused the destruction of his thumb-nail.

45

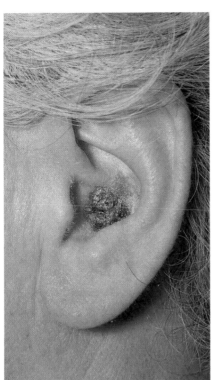

Fig. 86 Seborrhoeic warts are very common and are usually easy to diagnose, although sometimes if they are black in colour they can arouse suspicions of malignancy. They can be an annoying cosmetic problem. This oddly situated wart caused alarm, but a small biopsy confirmed its innocence and it was easily treated by cryotherapy.

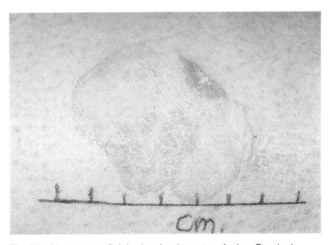

Fig. 87 A large superficial seborrhoeic wart on the leg. Surgical removal in this case could have produced a chronic ulcer, but it responded to light freezing.

46

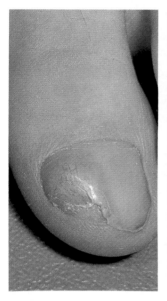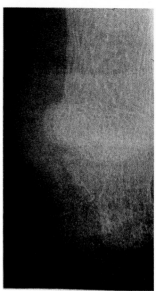

Fig. 88 Subungual fibromata secondary to exostoses are commonly misdiagnosed as warts. The correct diagnosis is important because the treatments are different. The X-ray accompanying this lesion is shown.

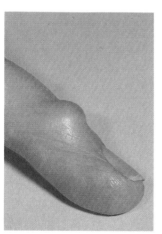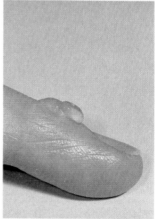

Fig. 89 Another common lump seen on the hands is the myxoma, or synovial cyst. This is seen over the terminal joints of the fingers, often in patients who have Heberden's nodes. On pricking the lump with a needle, material resembling glycerine can be expressed (right). Multiple punctures of such lesions are a simple and effective way of treating them.

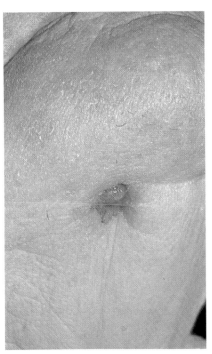

Fig. 90 A sinus track of dental origin. These are commonly referred to hospital as 'rodent ulcers'. The X-ray (below) shows the presence of dental infection. Treatment of this usually causes the skin lesion to heal up.

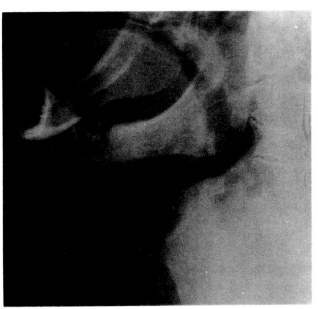

48

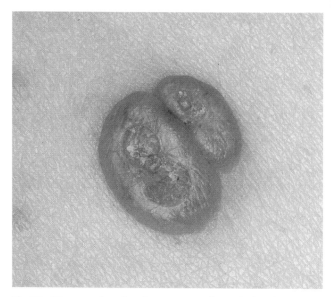

Fig. 91 Close-up view of molluscum contagiosum lesion showing characteristic umbilication. This is a viral infection and is interesting because it is frequently misdiagnosed, particulary when it occurs in adults. Destructive treatment is often a problem because the lesions may be widespread and often affect the face and eyelids in small children.

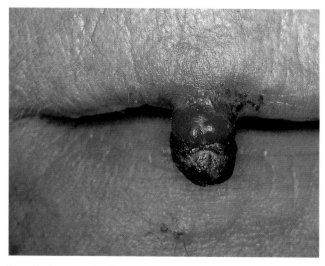

Fig. 92 An example of a pyogenic granuloma, which usually presents no treatment problem unless mistaken for malignant melanoma.

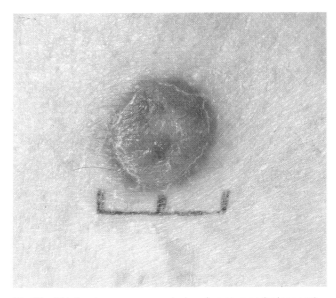

Fig. 93 A histiocytoma, a common lesion often seen on the legs and thighs, appearing for no apparent reason. Sometimes several are present. Characteristically they may be surmounted by a little brown pigment. This lesion is surrounded by brown pigment and this may arouse suspicion of malignancy.

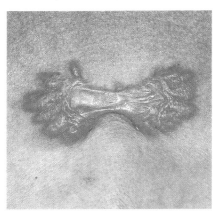

Fig. 94 Keloid occurring over the sternum. This butterfly or dumb-bell shape is characteristic. Treatment can be difficult and it should be remembered that surgery over the sternum or the deltoids may produce unsightly keloids in some patients.

When considering persistant lumps or irregularities in the skin, particularly in the middle-aged and elderly, it must be considered whether they are malignant or likely to become malignant. Actinic or senile keratoses are common, especially in those who have been exposed to excessive sunshine, even many years before.

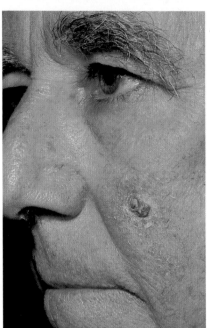

Fig. 95 A discrete warty lesion against a background of actinic change.

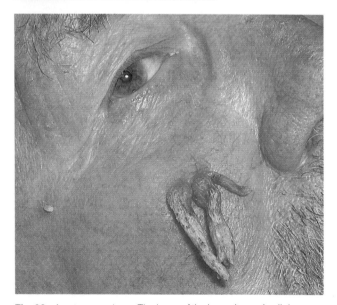

Fig. 96 A cutaneous horn. The base of the horn showed cellular irregularity but no actual invasion of the dermis.

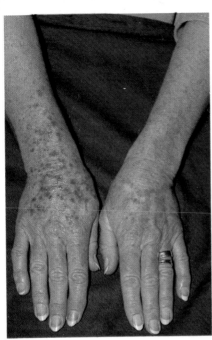

Fig. 97 Bilateral actinic changes. Those in the right hand have been exaggerated by the application of 5-fluorouracil ointment. This can be a useful treatment for this type of disorder as it shows up clinically unnoticeable areas of keratosis and enables large areas to be treated with relatively little discomfort.

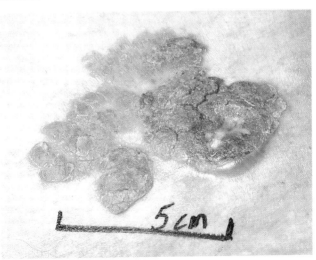

Fig. 98 A more specific type of premalignant lesion or intradermal cancer is Bowen's disease, which consists of defined erythematous scaly plaques often resembling psoriasis. In this patient the right side of the lesion has already undergone transformation into an invasive squamous-celled carcinoma.

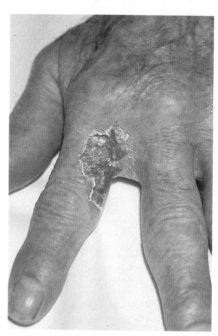

Fig. 99 Bowen's disease on the hand. This is quite common and can present diagnostic and therapeutic problems (compare Fig. 159).

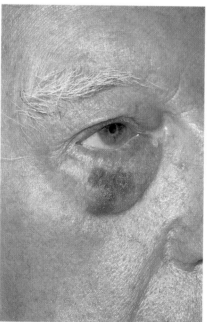

Fig. 100 Hutchinson's melanotic freckle, now more commonly known as lentigo meligna, although at this stage it is not actually malignant. See also Fig. 123.

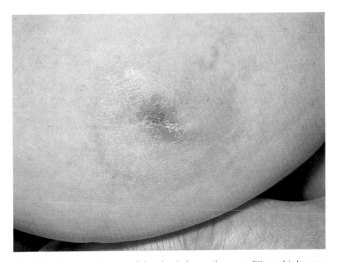

Fig. 101 Paget's disease of the nipple is another condition which may look deceptively innocent. This particular lesion had been declared benign on earlier clinical examination, but biopsy of the nipple showed Paget's disease. Any persisting 'eczema' involving the nipple should be regarded with the gravest suspicion if it does not clear up permanently and quickly with simple treatment.

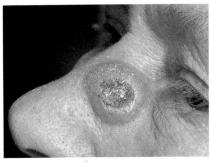
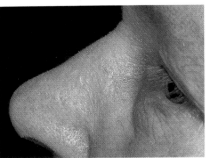

Fig. 102
Keratoacanthoma. These fairly common and important lesions can arise very rapidly, for which reason they were often regarded as highly malignant carcinomas. They are, in fact, benign and if left alone they disappear spontaneously, as in this case (below). Small biopsies are unhelpful as the histology of the benign keratoacanthoma closely resembles a malignant squamous-celled carcinoma. Where possible, the whole lesion should be removed surgically.

Squamous-celled carcinoma

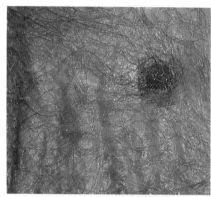

Fig. 103 An early squamous-celled carcinoma on the dorsum of the hand. Such lesions following actinic keratoses are relatively benign and seldom metastasise. However early diagnosis and treatment are essential because if neglected they may proceed to the appearance seen below.

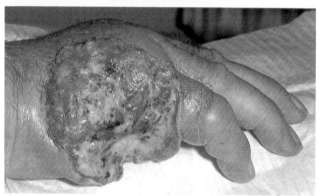

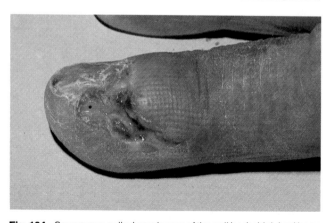

Fig. 104 Squamous-celled carcinoma of the nail bed which had been treated as an infection for three months.

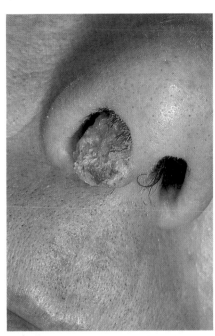

Fig. 105 Another squamous-celled carcinoma in an area which makes treatment difficult. Inadequate or superficial treatment of such lesions can be dangerous although they do not present much of a problem to modern surgeons.

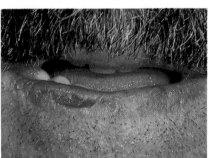

Fig. 106 A small superficial squamous-celled carcinoma of the lip (left) which is affected by actinic cheilitis. This can be treated by the simple operation of vermilionectomy. The cure rate is high and the cosmetic result can be excellent (below).

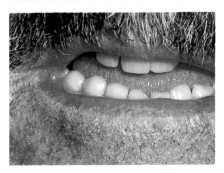

Basal cell carcinoma

This common condition is also known as rodent ulcer and is usually easy to recognise and treat. It is locally invasive and does not metastasise.

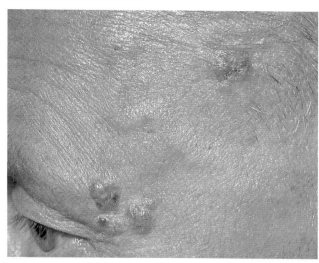

Fig. 107 These typically situated lesions are not ulcerated but show a characteristic translucent appearance with telangiectases on the surface.

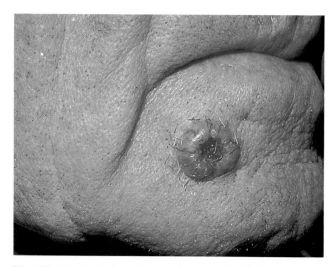

Fig. 108 A typical lesion with a rolled edge on the chin. Small vessels are seen to sweep over the edge and the centre is ulcerated.

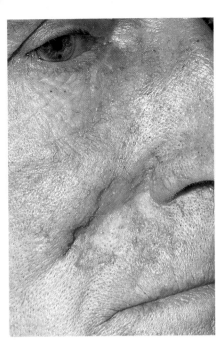

Fig. 109 A basal cell carcinoma presenting as a 'scar' with a defined edge. Sometimes ulcerated rodent ulcers do heal, but in this case ulceration had never occurred.

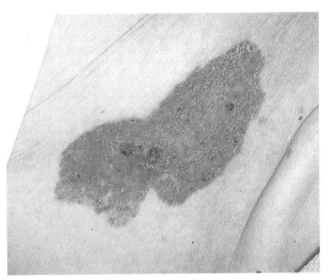

Fig. 110 Superficial basal cell carcinoma in situ in the epidermis. These lesions are often multiple on the trunk and are often disregarded as benign. Their malignant potential is low although some do eventually become deeply invasive.

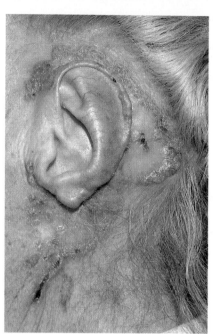

Fig. 111 A very extensive basal cell carcinoma. Not only is the skin attached to the skull but the pinna and external auditory meatus are involved.

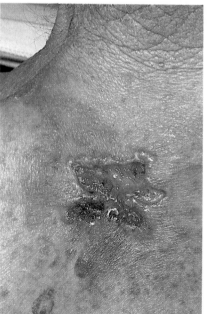

Fig. 112 Although most rodent ulcers occur on exposed areas they can also appear in areas which are usually covered, even in patients who have not been exposed to the sun.

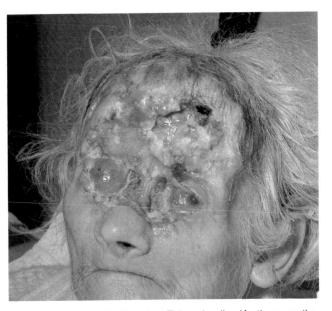

Fig. 113 A neglected rodent ulcer. This patient lived for three months after this picture was taken.

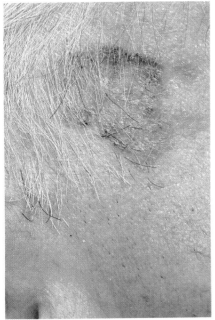

Fig. 114 Rodent ulcers can occur in the scalp and they may be pigmented.

Melanoma

Although much less common than squamous or basal-celled carcinoma, a melanoma rightly gives rise to much alarm. In recent years, proper prospective studies have been made of these lesions and there is increased knowledge about their behaviour. They are becoming much more common in Western countries and their incidence is closely related to sun exposure.

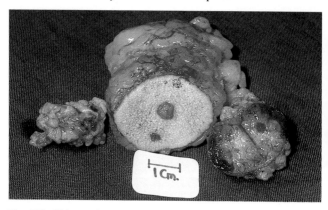

Fig. 115 This specimen shows a 3mm pigmented lesion from the buttock of a 23-year old woman who was waiting to see a surgeon about her bilateral inguinal herniae. There is pigmented enlargement of both inguinal nodes, and investigations showed the para-aortic glands to be involved. She died within three months.

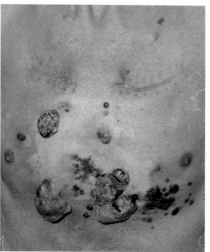

Fig. 116 Late result of metastasing malignant melanoma. This patient had lived quite happily with his secondaries for two years, until he was treated by cytotoxic drugs and was dead within a month.

61

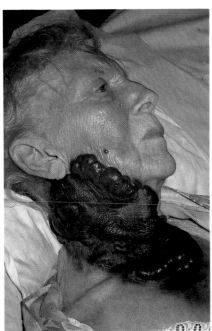

Fig. 117 A remarkable spreading melanoma on the neck of a 90-year old lady.

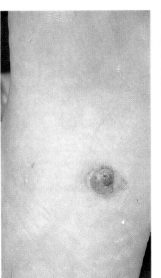 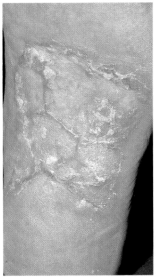

Fig. 118 Small pigmented lesion on the sole of the foot of the type known as superficial spreading melanoma (left). On the right is the result of a large skin graft following extensive excision.

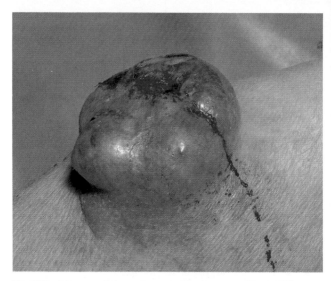

Fig. 119 A large nodular melanoma of the forearm with very little pigment. This lesion was excised but in such cases routine pre-operative chest X-rays should be ordered in case there are any secondary deposits.

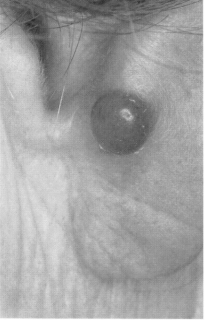

Fig. 120 A benign-looking, jet-black lesion on the lobe of the ear. In spite of removal of a large part of the ear this patient died of secondary deposits in the brain.

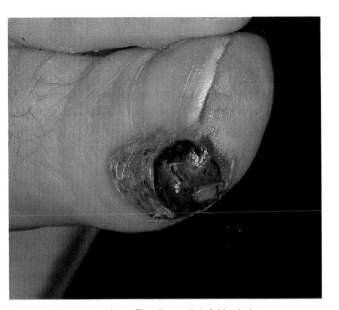

Fig. 121 Melanotic whitlow. The diagnosis is fairly obvious –
Characteristic pigment is usually seen.

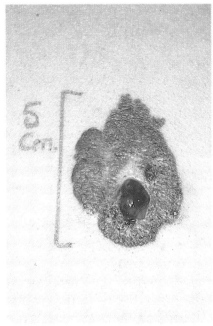

Fig. 122 Superficial
spreading melanoma
– one of the
commonest
presentations. This
long-standing black
and brown lesion had
recently developed a
nodule which is
ulcerated.

64

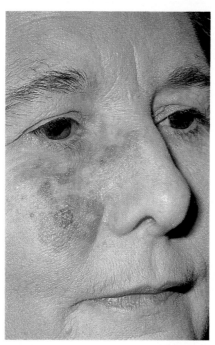

Fig. 123 Lentigo meligna melanoma. Two or three malignant nodules are present in a pre-existing melanotic freckle.

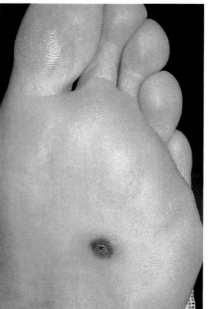

Fig. 124 This simple haematoma was mistaken for a melanoma (as in Fig. 118) and the surgeon was about to excise and graft it. A nick with a scapel blade expressed the contents of the haematoma and brought about a cure.

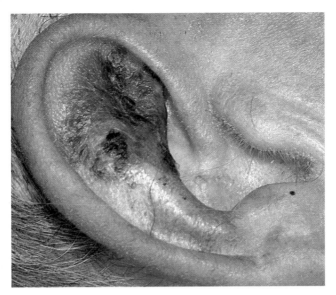

Fig. 125 This was referred as a malignant melanoma. A small punch biopsy was enough to show that the lesion was a harmless seborrhoeic wart. After two treatments with liquid nitrogen spray this lesion disappeared satisfactorily.

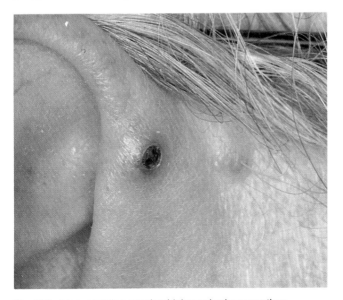

Fig. 126 A large senile comedo which required no more than expression of its contents.

66

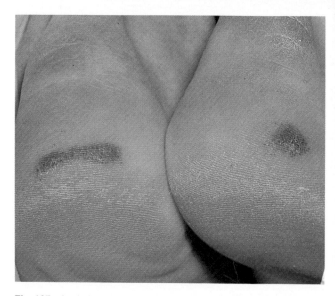

Fig. 127 A relatively common condition known as talon noir, which occurs on the heels of athletic people such as footballers and squash players. It is caused by blood pigment in the skin and results from a sudden shearing stress. The diagnosis is very obvious when it occurs on both feet. The lesions have a characteristic speckled appearance.

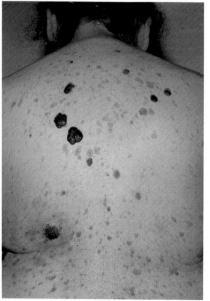

Fig. 128 Multiple seborrhoeic warts, some of which are pigmented and are jet-black. One wart at waist level has been irritated by a corset. These can often be mistaken for malignant melanomata.

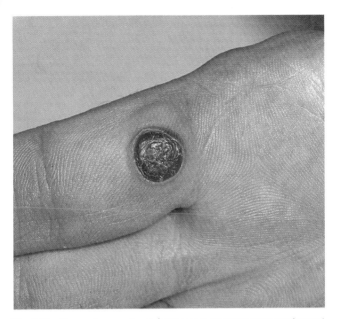

Fig. 129 Pyogenic granuloma. In this case, no biopsy was performed and the surgeon amputated the finger at the metacarpophalangeal joint.

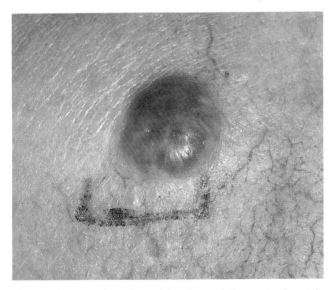

Fig. 130 Haemangioma. An excision biopsy confirmed the diagnosis and cured the condition.

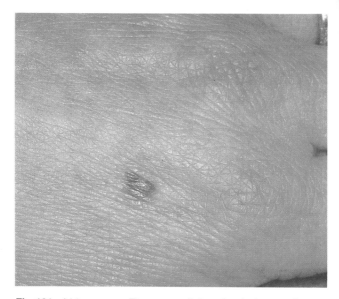

Fig. 131 A blue naevus. These normally harmless lesions can be difficult to diagnose.

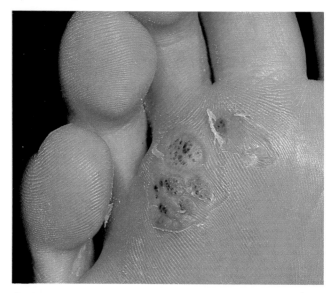

Fig. 132 Resolving plantar warts. This black appearance is characteristic and indicates that they will disappear in a short time. These were, however, referred as malignant melanomata although malignant melanoma before puberty is excessively rare.

Erythematous and Bullous Disorders

Apart from the common fevers of childhood, erythematous eruptions are common and may present diagnostic difficulties.

Fig. 133 An acute allergic sensitivity to penicillin.

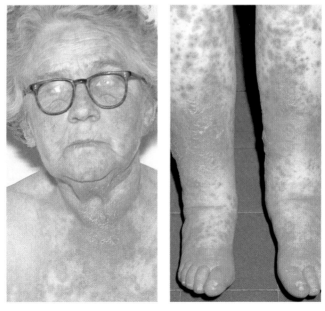

Fig. 134 Extensive erythema due to phenylbutazone, which is becoming bullous on the legs.

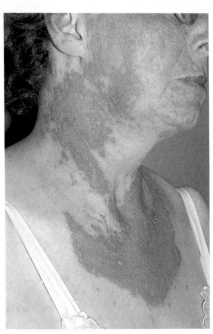

Fig. 135 Erythematous light sensitive reaction to a drug – in this case an antimalarial given for rheumatoid arthritis.

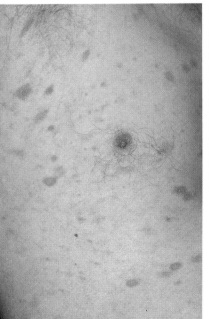

Fig. 136 Most of these erythematous, morbilliform and bullous eruptions are non-specific – that is, a similar type of rash can be caused by a wide variety of drugs. Some drugs, however, produce a distinctive pattern. For example gold, used in rheumatoid arthritis, may produce a rash resembling pityriasis rosea (see Fig. 145).

71

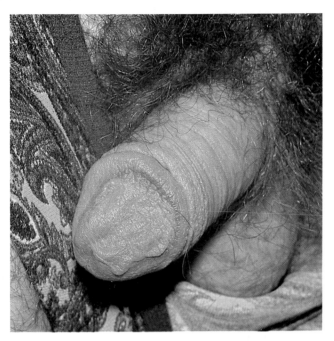

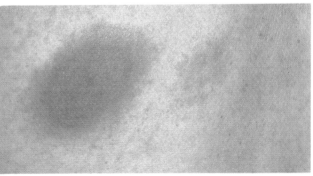

Fig. 137 A fixed drug eruption. Sometimes the lesion is single but occasionally three or four may be present. They can occur anywhere on the skin surface but are particularly common around the mouth and genitalia. There is a long list of drugs which can cause such an eruption – the commonest used to be phenolphthalein, used as a laxative. Tetracyclines are perhaps the commonest cause now although this example was caused by non-steroidal anti-inflammatory drugs. All sorts of odd substances can occasionally cause this eruption, such as quinine in soft drinks and coloured icing on cakes! Since this is a harmless eruption it is one of the few types of drug reaction which can be tested by giving provocative doses of the suspected drug.

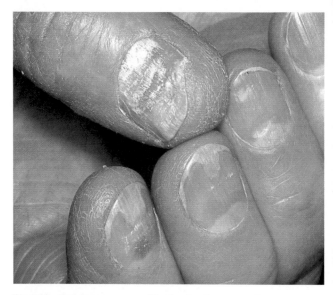

Fig. 138 Nail damage caused by the drug benoxaprofen, now withdrawn. Similar reactions may occur with tetracyclines, particularly demethylchlortetracycline.

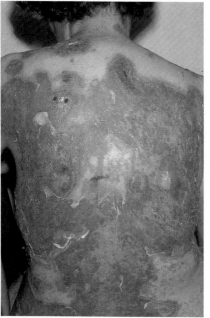

Fig. 139 Pemphigus foliaceus type of reaction, characteristically caused by penicillamine, used in treating rheumatoid arthritis. Rheumatoid arthritis is a distressing enough illness in its own right and most of the second and third line drugs used in its treatment can cause unpleasant skin reactions.

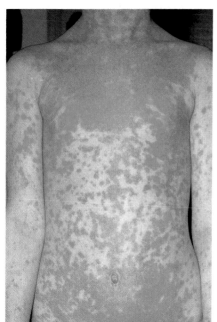

Fig. 140 Characteristic widespread morbilliform reaction which may be due to the original throat infection or to the ampicillin used to treat it.

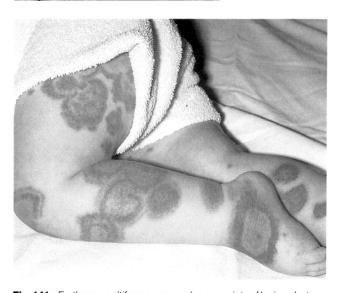

Fig. 141 Erythema multiforme can produce a variety of lesions but particularly these ringed or iris lesions. Although seen here in a baby, it is much more common in older children or adults. It is often recurrent and may follow herpes simplex or other virus infections.

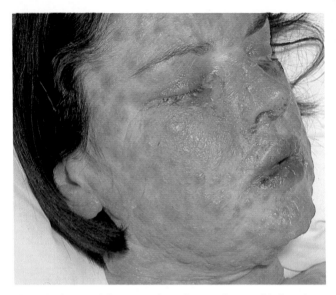

Fig. 142 Stevens Johnson syndrome is a term best avoided or at least not misused as a synonym for erythema multiforme. It should only be used when there is eye involvement.

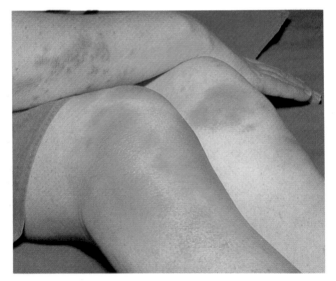

Fig. 143 Erythema nodosum. Characteristic fiery red, infiltrated lesions are seen on the knees and legs and also on the arms. Such patients require a battery of investigations to exclude the various systemic concomitants of this condition.

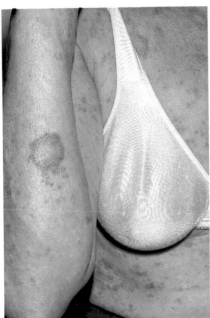

Fig. 144 Pityriasis rosea (see Fig. 136) may be a reaction to gold, but the spontaneously occurring form is much more common. This patient has a herald patch on the right fore-arm which had been diagnosed as ringworm before the appearance of a generalised eruption.

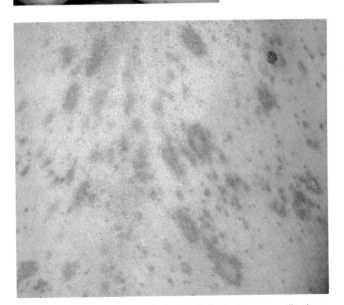

Fig. 145 Pityriasis rosaea on the back with the lesions spreading in a characteristic way, roughly along the lines of the ribs. Many lesions show characteristic peripheral centripetal scaling.

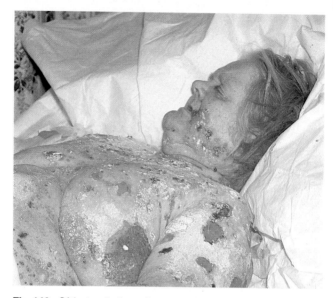

Fig. 146 Of the true bullous diseases, pemphigus vulgaris is fortunately relatively uncommon in Britain. It is a distressing condition which is fatal unless treated, and the treatment itself is not without risk.

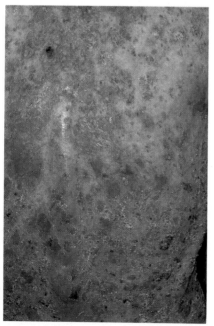

Fig. 147 Pemphigus foliaceus on the back. This condition cleared dramatically with relatively small doses of steroids.

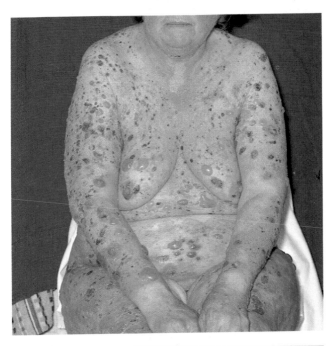

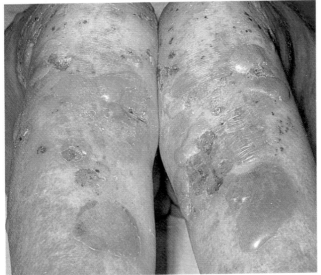

Fig. 148 Bullous pemphigoid. This is much more common then pemphigus vulgaris. Large bullae are seen on the legs, many arising from normal skin.

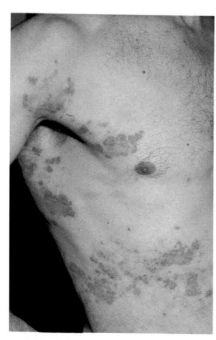

Fig. 149 Before treating the bullous disorders it is important to make a precise diagnosis by routine and immune histological investigation. This is especially true in dermatitis herpetiformis. This eruption is characteristic and rather eczema-like and is accompanied by intense itching.

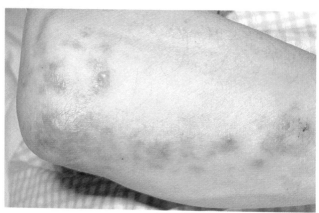

Fig. 150 This example of dermatitis herpetiformis shows vesicles. Many patients do not show vesicles, or they are only seen occasionally during the course of the illness, which may persist for the rest of the patient's life. Although this condition normally responds to dapsone or other sulphonamide drugs, this should not be used as a sole diagnostic criterion, since other conditions will also respond to these drugs. Proper histological diagnosis should be made, including demonstration of IgA and jejunal biopsy. A gluten-free diet may be indicated.

These blistering conditions are all relatively uncommon compared, that is, with the blisters seen in the various forms of eczema, drug eruption etc. Although pemphigus and pemphigoid do occur in childhood, they are very rare.

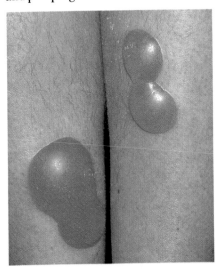

Fig. 151 Large blisters on the shins which were referred to a clinic as pemphigus. They were, in fact, simply the result of an allergic reaction to insect bites.

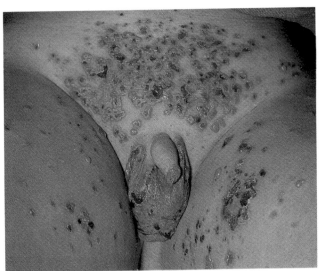

Fig. 152 Chronic bullous disease of childhood. This is a rare condition and characteristically produces blisters around the genitalia, thighs and lower abdomen. It is usually controlled by sulphapyridine, but remits after months or even years.

Fungal Diseases of the Skin

These conditions are frequently misdiagnosed, and are much less common in temperate climates than is commonly believed.

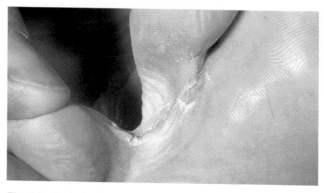

Fig. 153 Typical mild athlete's foot, tinea pedis. Not all interdigital rashes are tinea; many are due to simple maceration, and even psoriasis can present in this manner. In the outer toe space, a soft corn may mimic tinea. The treatment is never urgent and can readily await microscopic or cultural identification.

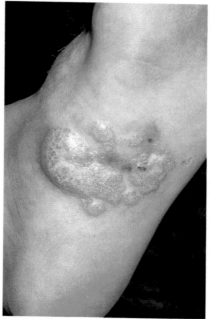

Fig. 154 Blistering form of tinea pedis (compare with contact dermatitis due to rubber footwear, Fig. 26).

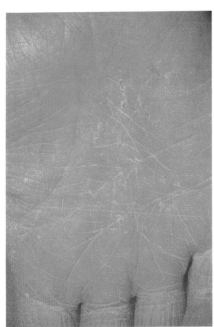

Fig. 155 Tinea does not produce interdigital lesions between the fingers as it does on the foot. When fungal infections attack the hands, they more commonly produce a dry, scaly appearance of the skin creases.

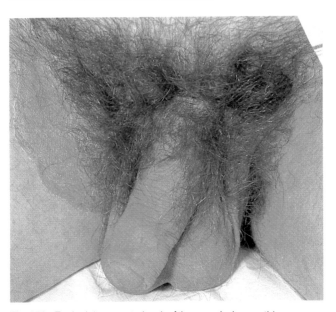

Fig. 156 Typical demarcated rash of tinea cruris. In men this commonly affects the left groin more than the right.

82

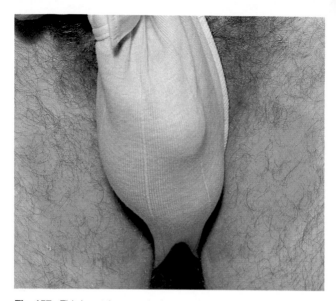

Fig. 157 This is not tinea cruris due to a dermatophyte fungus, but is an example of erythrasma. This is a quite different condition requiring antibiotic treatment, not fungicides.

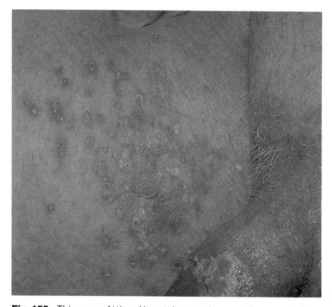

Fig. 158 This case of 'tinea' is not due to a ringworm fungus – but to *Candida albicans*.

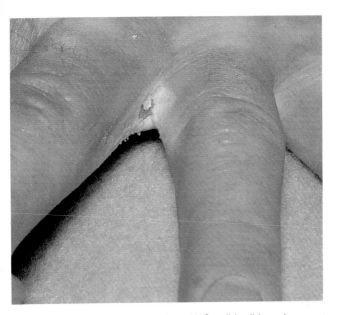

Fig. 159 A fairly uncommon infection with *Candida albicans* known as *Erosio blastomycetica interdigitalis* (compare Fig. 99).

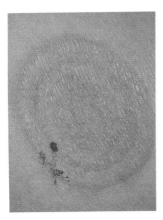

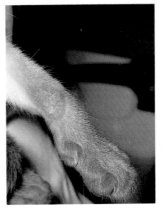

Fig. 160 This patient shows 'rings' but this is not a common presentation of a fungal infection. Discoid or circular lesions are more commonly due to psoriasis or eczema. This type of tinea is usually caused by infection by an animal fungus; here from a cat.

Fig. 161 The pets which transmit ringworm should also be examined and treated. Cats are probably the most common vectors in the UK, although in rural areas, cattle are also vectors.

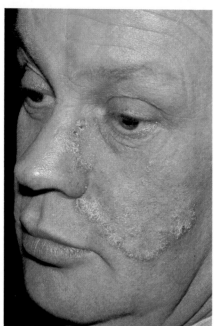

Fig. 162 A patient showing a lesion with a circinate outline. It is tinea, but the patient was a psoriatic and the infection had provoked psoriasis. Griseofulvin cleared both the ringworm and psoriasis.

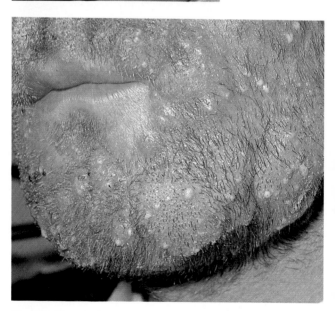

Fig. 163 Tinea barbae. This and other pustular forms of ringworm are commonly missed and treated as pyococcal infections or carbuncles.

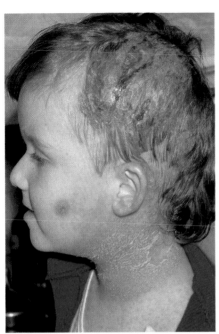

Fig. 164 Pustular ringworm or kerion of a child's scalp which had been neglected. The child suffered permanent alopecia as a result.

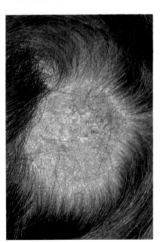

Fig. 165 Classical form of small-spored ringworm of the scalp. A well-demarcated partly bald patch shows broken-off stumps of hair which fluoresce vividly under Wood's light. This is now an uncommon condition

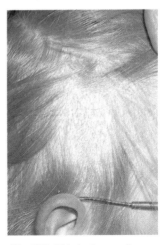

Fig. 166 This is also small-spored ringworm, but looks more like diffuse seborrhoea capitis.

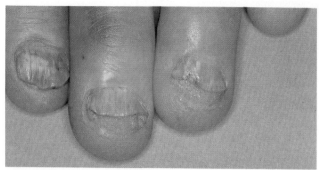

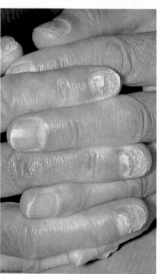

Fig. 167 Ringworm of the nails. As is often the case, this is unilateral. A clinical diagnosis of ringworm of the nails is not possible as it can closely resemble psoriasis, eczema or occupational or traumatic dermatitis. Microscopic and preferably cultural confirmation is needed before the necessarily long treatment with griseofulvin is begun.

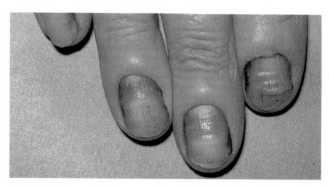

Fig. 168 Characteristic paronychia and onychia due to *Candida albicans* with pigmentation due to bacterial infection.

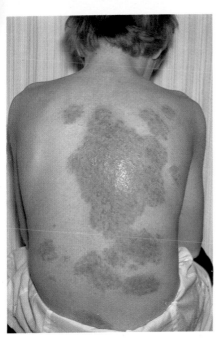

Fig. 169 Extensive ringworm of animal origin on a child's back, which could be mistaken for psoriasis.

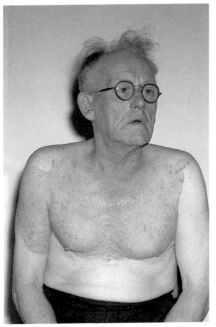

Fig. 170 Extensive tinea on the trunk. Note the clearly demarcated edge and the curious distribution on the upper chest.

88

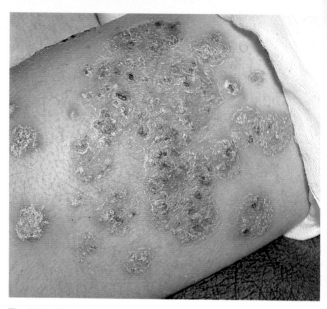

Fig. 171 Tinea after treatment with powerful topical steroids. This is often termed tinea incognita.

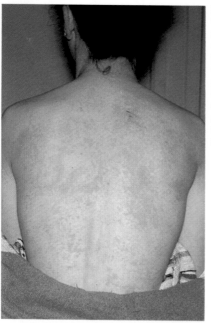

Fig. 172 Tinea versicolor. This may sometimes appear as dark patches on a pale skin or vice-versa. Wood's lamp examination can help in making the diagnosis, but it is sometimes difficult to exclude vitiligo, or even pityriasis alba.

Index

All entries refer to Fig. numbers